The Definitive Keto Chaffle Cookbook Recipes for Beginners

The Ultimate Recipes to Taste the Best Keto Meals and Enjoy your Diet

Veronica Lang

Table of contents

Red Velvet Chaffle

Servings: 3

Cooking Time: 12 Minutes

Ingredients:

1 egg

¼ cup mozzarella cheese, shredded 1 oz. cream cheese

4 tablespoons almond flour 1 teaspoon baking powder 2 teaspoons sweetener

1   teaspoon red velvet extract

2   tablespoons cocoa powder

Directions:

1.   Combine all the ingredients in a bowl.

2.   Plug in your waffle maker.

3.   Pour some of the batter into the waffle maker.

4.   Seal and cook for minutes.

5.   Open and transfer to a plate.

6. Repeat the steps with the remaining batter. Nutrition value:

Calories 126 Fat 10.1g Carbohydrate 6.5g Protein 5.9g Sugars 0.2g

Walnuts Lowcarb Chaffles

Servings: 2

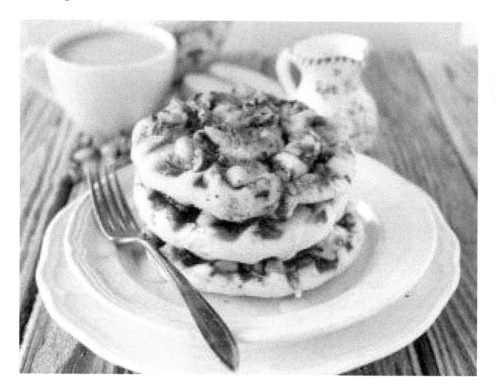

Cooking Time:5 minutes

Ingredients:

2 tbsps. cream cheese

½ tsp almonds flour

¼ tsp. baking powder 1 large egg

¼ cup chopped walnuts

Pinch of stevia extract powder

Directions:

1.   Preheat your waffle maker.

2.   Spray waffle maker with cooking spray.

3.   In a bowl, add cream cheese, almond flour, baking powder, egg, walnuts, and stevia.

4.   Mix all ingredients,

5.   Spoon walnut batter in the waffle maker and cook for about 2-3 minutes.

6.   Let chaffles cool at room temperature before serving. Nutrition value per Servings:

Calories 170 Fat: 13 g ; Carbs: 2 g ; Protein: 11 g

Beginner Brownies Chaffle

Servings: 2

Cooking Time:5 minutes

Ingredients:

1 cup cheddar cheese 1 tbsp. cocoa powder

½ tsp baking powder 1 large egg.

¼ cup melted keto chocolate chips for topping

Directions:

1.   Preheat dash minutesi waffle iron and grease it.

2.   Blend all ingredients in a blender until mixed.

3.   Pour 1 tsp. cheese in a waffle maker and then pour the mixture in the center of greased waffle.

4.   Again sprinkle cheese on the batter.

5.   Close the waffle maker.

6.   Cook chaffles for about 4-5 minutes until cooked and crispy.

7.   Once chaffles are cooked remove.

8.	Top with melted chocolate and enjoy! Nutrition value per Servings:

Calories 170 Fat: 13 g ; Carbs: 2 g ; Protein: 11 g

Holidays Chaffles

Servings:4

Cooking Time:5minutes

Ingredients:

1   cup egg whites

2   tsps. coconut flour ½ tsp.vanilla 1 tsp. baking powder

1 tsp. baking soda

1/8 tsp cinnamon powder

1 cup mozzarella cheese, grated TOPPING:

Cranberries

keto Chocolate sauce

Directions:

1.   Make 4 minutesi chaffles from the chaffle ingredients.

2.   Top with chocolate sauce and cranberries

3.   Serve hot and enjoy! Nutrition value per Servings:

Calories: 145 Fat: 9.4g Carbohydrates: 1g Sugar: 0.2g Protein: 14.3g

Cherry Chocolate Chaffle

Servings: 1

Cooking Time: 10 Minutes

Ingredients:

1 egg, lightly beaten

1 tbsp unsweetened chocolate chips 2 tbsp sugar-free cherry pie filling 2 tbsp heavy whipping cream

1/2 cup mozzarella cheese, shredded 1/2 tsp baking powder, gluten-free

1 tbsp Swerve

1   tbsp unsweetened cocoa powder 1 tbsp almond flour

Directions:

1.   Preheat the waffle maker.

2.   In a bowl, whisk together egg, cheese, baking powder, Swerve, cocoa powder, and almond flour.

3.   Spray waffle maker with cooking spray.

4.   Pour batter in the hot waffle maker and cook until golden brown.

5.　　Top with cherry pie filling, heavy whipping cream, and chocolate chips and serve.

Nutrition value:

Calories 2 Fat 22 g Carbohydrates 8.5 g Sugar 0.5 g Protein 12.7 g

Bacon, Egg & Avocado Chaffle Sandwich

Servings: 2

Cooking Time: 10 Minutes

Ingredients: Cooking spray 4 slices bacon

2   eggs

½ avocado, mashed

4 basic chaffles

2 leaves lettuce

Directions:

1.   Coat your skillet with cooking spray.

2.   Cook the bacon until golden and crisp.

3.   Transfer into a paper towel lined plate.

4.   Crack the eggs into the same pan and cook until firm.

5.   Flip and cook until the yolk is set.

6.   Spread the avocado on the chaffle.

7.   Top with lettuce, egg and bacon.

8.   Top with another chaffle. Nutrition value:

Calories 372 Fat 30.1g Carbohydrate 5.4g Sugars 0.6g Protein
20.6g

Crunchy Coconut Chaffles Cake

Servings:4

Cooking Time: 15 Minutes

Ingredients:

4 large eggs

1 cup shredded cheese 2 tbsps. coconut cream 2 tbsps. coconut flour. 1 tsp. stevia TOPPING

1 cup heavy cream 8 oz. raspberries

4 oz. blueberries

2 oz. cherries

Directions:

1.   Make 4 thin round chaffles with the chaffle ingredients. Once chaffles are cooked, set in layers on a plate.

2.   Spread heavy cream in each layer.

3.   Top with raspberries then blueberries and cherries.

4.   Serve and enjoy! Nutrition value per Servings:

Calories: 145 Fat: 9.4g Carbohydrates: 1g Sugar: 0.2g Protein: 14.3g

Coffee Flavored Chaffle

Servings:4

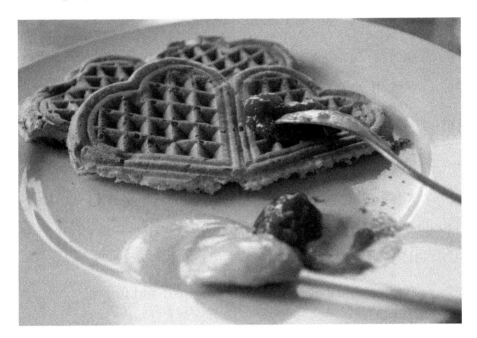

Cooking Time:7-9 Minutes

Ingredients:

Batter 4 eggs

4 ounces cream cheese

½ teaspoon vanilla extract

6 tablespoons strong boiled espresso

¼ cup stevia

½ cup almond flour

1   teaspoon baking powder Pinch of salt

Other

2   tablespoons butter to brush the waffle maker

Directions:

1.   Preheat the waffle maker.

2.   Add the eggs and cream cheese to a bowl and stir in the vanilla extract, espresso, stevia, almond flour, baking powder, and salt pinch.

3.   Stir just until everything is combined and fully incorporated.

4.   Brush the heated waffle maker with butter and add a few tablespoons of the batter.

5.   Close the lid and cook for about 7-8 minutes depending on your waffle maker.

6.   Serve and enjoy. Nutrition value per Servings:

Calories 300, fat 26.g, carbs 4.8 g, sugar 0.5 g, Protein 10.8 g

Italian Sausage Chaffles

Servings: 2

Cooking Time: 8 Minutes

Ingredients:

1 egg, beaten

1 cup cheddar cheese, shredded

¼ cup Parmesan cheese, grated 1 lb. Italian sausage, crumbled 2 teaspoons baking powder

1 cup almond flour

Directions:

1.   Preheat your waffle maker.

2.   Mix all the ingredients in a bowl.

3.   Pour half of the mixture into the waffle maker.

4.   Cover and cook for minutes.

5.   Transfer to a plate.

6.   Let cool to make it crispy.

7.   Do the same steps to make the next chaffle. Nutrition value:

Calories 332 Fat 27.1g Carbohydrate 1.9g Sugars 0.1g Protein 19.6g

Chaffles With Strawberry Frosty

Servings:2

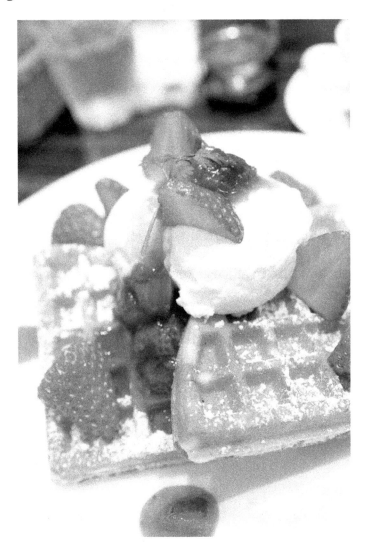

Cooking Time: 5 Minutes

Ingredients:

1 cup frozen strawberries

1/2 cup Heavy cream

1 tsp stevia

1 scoop protein powder

3 keto chaffles

Directions:

1.   Mix all ingredients in a mixing bowl.

2.   Pour mixture in silicone molds and freeze in a freezer for about 4 hours to set.

3.   Once frosty is set, top on keto chaffles and enjoy!
Nutrition value per Servings:

Calories: 145 Fat: 9.4g Carbohydrates: 1g Sugar: 0.2g Protein: 14.3g

Hot Chocolate Breakfast Chaffle

Servings: 2

Cooking Time: 14 Minutes

Ingredients:

1   egg, beaten

2   tbsp almond flour

1 tbsp unsweetened cocoa powder 2 tbsp cream cheese, softened

¼ cup finely grated Monterey Jack cheese 2 tbsp sugar-free maple syrup

1 tsp vanilla extract

Directions:

1.   Preheat the waffle iron.

2.   In a medium bowl, mix all the ingredients.

3.   Open the iron, lightly grease with cooking spray and pour in half of the mixture.

4.   Close the iron and cook until crispy, 7 minutes.

5.   Remove the chaffle onto a plate and set aside.

6.   Pour the remaining batter in the iron and make the second chaffle.

7.   Allow cooling and serve afterward. Nutrition value per Servings:

Calories 47 Fats 3.67g Carbs 1.39g Protein 2.29g

Pecan Pumpkin Chaffle

Servings: 2

Cooking Time: 15 Minutes

Ingredients:

1   egg

2   tbsp pecans, toasted and chopped

2 tbsp almond flour 1 tsp erythritol

1/4 tsp pumpkin pie spice 1 tbsp pumpkin puree

1/2 cup mozzarella cheese, grated

Directions:

1.   Preheat your waffle maker.

2.   Beat egg in a small bowl.

3.   Add remaining ingredients and mix well.

4.   Spray waffle maker with cooking spray.

5.   Pour half batter in the hot waffle maker and cook for minutes or until golden brown. Repeat with the remaining batter.

6.   Serve and enjoy. Nutrition value:

Calories 121Fat 9.g Carbohydrates 5.7 g Sugar 3.3 g Protein 6.7 g

Swiss Bacon Chaffle

Servings: 2

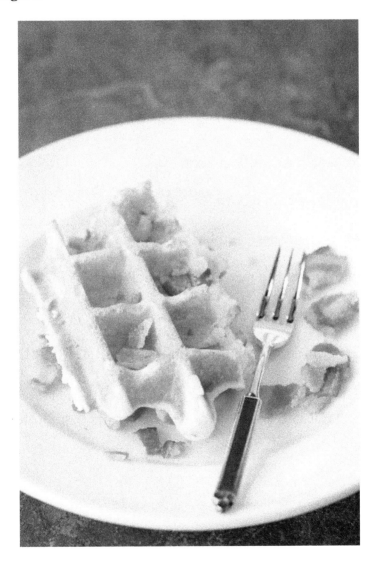

Cooking Time: 8 Minutes

Ingredients:

1   egg

½ cup Swiss cheese

2   tablespoons cooked crumbled bacon

Directions:

1.   Preheat your waffle maker.

2.   Beat the egg in a bowl.

3.   Stir in the cheese and bacon.

4.   Pour half of the mixture into the device.

5.   Close and cook for 4 minutes.

6.   Cook the second chaffle using the same steps. Nutrition value:

Calories 23 Fat 17.6g Carbohydrate 1.9g Sugars 0.5g Protein 17.1g

Bacon, Olives & Cheddar Chaffle

Servings: 2

Cooking Time: 8 Minutes

Ingredients:

1 egg

½ cup cheddar cheese, shredded

1 tablespoon black olives, chopped 1 tablespoon bacon bits
Directions:

1.   Plug in your waffle maker.

2.   In a bowl, beat the egg and stir in the cheese.

3.   Add the black olives and bacon bits.

4.   Mix well.

5.   Add half of the mixture into the waffle maker.

6.   Cover and cook for 4 minutes.

7.   Open and transfer to a plate.

8.   Let cool for 2 minutes.

9. Cook the other chaffle using the remaining batter.

Nutrition value:

Calories 202 Fat 16g Carbohydrate 0.9g Protein 13.4g Sugars 0.3g

Breakfast Spinach Ricotta Chaffles

Servings: 4

Cooking Time: 28 Minutes

Ingredients:

4 oz frozen spinach, thawed, squeezed dry 1 cup ricotta cheese

2 eggs, beaten

½ tsp garlic powder

¼ cup finely grated Pecorino Romano cheese

½ cup finely grated mozzarella cheese

Salt and freshly ground black pepper to taste

Directions:

1.   Preheat the waffle iron.

2.   In a medium bowl, mix all the ingredients.

3.   Open the iron, lightly grease with cooking spray and spoon in a quarter of the mixture.

4.   Close the iron and cook until brown and crispy, 7 minutes.

5. Remove the chaffle onto a plate and set aside.

6. Make three more chaffles with the remaining mixture.

7. Allow cooling and serve afterward. Nutrition value:

Calories 50 Fat 13.15g Carbs 5.06g Protein 12.79g

Pumpkin Chaffle With Frosting

Servings: 2

Cooking Time: 15 Minutes

Ingredients:

1 egg, lightly beaten

1   tbsp sugar-free pumpkin puree 1/4 tsp pumpkin pie spice 1/2 cup mozzarella cheese, shredded For frosting:

1/2 tsp vanilla 2 tbsp Swerve

2   tbsp cream cheese, softened

Directions:

1.   Preheat your waffle maker.

2.   Add egg in a bowl and whisk well.

3.   Add pumpkin puree, pumpkin pie spice, and cheese and stir well.

4.   Spray waffle maker with cooking spray.

5.   Pour 1/2 of the batter in the hot waffle maker and cook for 3-4 minutes or until golden brown. Repeat with the remaining batter.

6.   In a small bowl, mix all frosting ingredients until smooth.

7.   Add frosting on top of hot chaffles and serve. Nutrition value:

Calories 97 Carbohydrates 3.6 g Sugar 0.6 g Protein 5.6 g

Thanksgiving Pumpkin Latte With Chaffles

Servings: 1

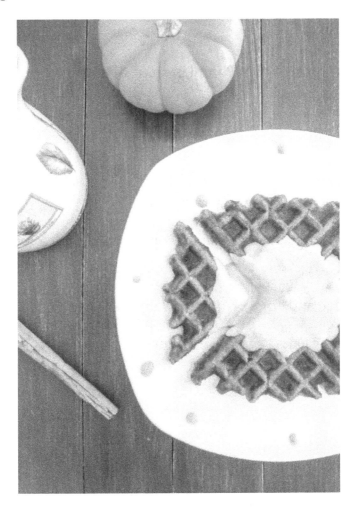

Cooking Time:5minutes

Ingredients:

3/4 cup unsweetened coconut milk 2 tbsps. Heavy cream

2 tbsps. Pumpkin puree 1 tsp. stevia

1/4 tsp pumpkin spice 1/4 tsp Vanilla extract 1/4 cup espresso
FOR TOPPING:

2 scoop whipped cream Pumpkin spice 2 heart shape minutesi chaffles Directions:

1.   Mix all recipe ingredients in mug and microwave for minutesute.

2.   Pour thelatte intoa serving glass.

3.   Top with a heavy cream scoop, pumpkin spice, and chaffle.

4.   Serve and enjoy! Nutrition value per Servings:

Calories: 145 Fat: 9.4g Carbohydrates: 1g Sugar: 0.2g Protein: 14.3g

Choco And Strawberries Chaffles

Servings: 2

Cooking Time:5 minutes

Ingredients:

1   tbsp. almond flour

1/2 cup strawberry puree 1/2 cup cheddar cheese 1 tbsp. cocoa powder

½ tsp baking powder 1 large egg.

2   tbsps. coconut oil. melted 1/2 tsp vanilla extract optional
Directions:

1.   Preheat waffle iron while you are mixing the ingredients.

2.   Melt oil in a microwave.

3.   In a small mixing bowl, mix flour, baking powder, flour, and vanilla until well.

4.   Add egg, melted oil, ½ cup cheese and strawberry puree tothe flour mixture.

5.   Pour 1/8 cup cheese in a waffle maker and then pour the mixture in the greased waffle center.

6.   Again sprinkle cheese on the batter.

7.   Close the waffle maker.

8.   Cook chaffles for about 4-5 minutes until cooked and crispy.

9.   Once chaffles are cooked,remove and enjoy! Nutrition value per Servings:

Calories: 145 Fat: 9.4g Carbohydrates: 1g Sugar: 0.2g Protein: 14.3g

Lemon And Paprika Chaffles

Servings: 4

Cooking Time: 28 Minutes

Ingredients:

1 egg, beaten

1 oz cream cheese, softened

1/3 cup finely grated mozzarella cheese 1 tbsp almond flour

1 tsp butter, melted

1 tsp maple (sugar-free) syrup ½ tsp sweet paprika

½ tsp lemon extract

Directions:

1.   Preheat the waffle iron.

2.   Mix all the ingredients in a medium bowl

3.   Open the iron and pour in a quarter of the mixture. Close and cook until crispy, 7 minutes.

4.   Remove the chaffle onto a plate and make 3 more with the remaining mixture.

5. Cut each chaffle into wedges, plate, allow cooling and serve. Nutrition value:

Calories 48 Fats 4.22g Carbs 8 Protein 2g

Triple Chocolate Chaffle

Servings:4

Cooking Time:7-9 Minutes

Ingredients:

Batter 4 eggs

4 ounces cream cheese, softened

1 ounce dark unsweetened chocolate, melted 1 teaspoon vanilla extract

5 tablespoons almond flour 3 tablespoons cocoa powder

1½ teaspoons baking powder

¼ cup dark unsweetened chocolate chips

2 tablespoons butter to brush the waffle maker

Directions:

1.   Preheat the waffle maker.

2.   Add the eggs and cream cheese to a bowl and stir with a wire whisk until just combined.

3.   Add the vanilla extract and mix until combined.

4.   Stir in the almond flour, cocoa powder, and baking powder and mix until combined.

5.   Add the chocolate chips and stir.

6.   Brush the heated waffle maker with butter and add a few tablespoons of the batter.

7.   Close the lid and cook for about 8 minutes depending on your waffle maker.

8.   Serve and enjoy. Nutrition value per Servings:

Calories 385, fat 33 g, carbs 10.6 g, sugar 0.7 g, Protein 12.g,

Mixed Berry-Vanilla Chaffles

Servings: 4

Cooking Time: 28 Minutes

Ingredients:

1 egg, beaten

½ cup finely grated mozzarella cheese 1 tbsp cream cheese, softened

1   tbsp sugar-free maple syrup 2 strawberries, sliced

2   raspberries, slices

¼ tsp blackberry extract

¼ tsp vanilla extract

½ cup plain yogurt for serving

Directions:

1.   Preheat the waffle iron.

2.   In a medium bowl, mix all the ingredients except the yogurt.

3.   Open the iron, lightly grease with cooking spray and pour in a quarter of the mixture.

4.   Close the iron and cook until golden brown and crispy, 7 minutes.

5.   Remove the chaffle onto a plate and set aside.

6.   Make three more chaffles with the remaining mixture.

7.   To Servings: top with the yogurt and enjoy. Nutrition value per Servings:

Calories 75 Carbs 12g Protein 4.5g Sugar 0.5g

Nut Butter Chaffle

Servings: 2

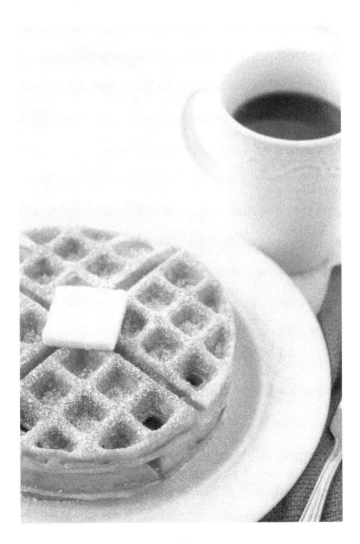

Cooking Time: 8 Minutes

Ingredients:

1 egg

½ cup mozzarella cheese, shredded 2 tablespoons almond flour

½ teaspoon baking powder 1 tablespoon sweetener

1   teaspoon vanilla

2   tablespoons nut butter

Directions:

1.   Turn on the waffle maker.

2.   Beat the egg in a bowl and combine with the cheese.

3.   In another bowl, mix the almond flour, baking powder and sweetener.

4.   In the third bowl, blend the vanilla extract and nut butter.

5.   Gradually add the almond flour mixture into the egg mixture.

6.   Then, stir in the vanilla extract.

7.   Pour the batter into the waffle maker.

8. Cook for 4 minutes.

9. Transfer to a plate and let cool for 2 minutes.

10. Repeat the steps with the remaining batter. Nutrition value:

Calories 168 Fat 15.5g Carbohydrate 1.6g Protein 5.4g Sugars 0.6g

Keto Coffee Chaffles

Servings: 2

Cooking Time:5 minutes

Ingredients:

1 tbsp. almond flour 1 tbsp. instant coffee

1/2 cup cheddar cheese

½ tsp baking powder 1 large egg Directions:

1.   Preheat waffle iron and grease with cooking spray

2.   Meanwhile, in a small mixing bowl, mix all ingredients and ½ cup cheese.

3.   Pour 1/8 cup cheese in a waffle maker and then pour the mixture in the greased waffle center.

4.   Again, sprinkle cheese on the batter.

5.   Close the waffle maker.

6.   Cook chaffles for about 4-5 minutes until cooked and crispy.

7.   Once chaffles are cooked, remove and enjoy! Nutrition value per Servings:

Calories: 145 Fat: 9.4g Carbohydrates: 1g Sugar: 0.2g Protein: 14.3g

Scrambled Egg Stuffed Chaffles

Servings: 4

Cooking Time: 28 Minutes

Ingredients:

For the chaffles:

1 cup finely grated cheddar cheese 2 eggs, beaten

For the egg stuffing:

1 tbsp olive oil

1 small red bell pepper 4 large eggs

1 small green bell pepper

Salt and freshly ground black pepper to taste 2 tbsp grated Parmesan cheese

Directions:

1.   For the chaffles:

2.   Preheat the waffle iron.

3.   In a medium bowl, mix the cheddar cheese and egg.

4. Open the iron, pour in a quarter of the mixture, close, and cook until crispy, 6 to 7 minutes.

5. Plate and make three more chaffles using the remaining mixture.

6. For the egg stuffing:

7. Meanwhile, heat the olive oil in a medium skillet over medium heat on a stovetop.

8. In a medium bowl, beat the eggs with the bell peppers, salt, black pepper, and Parmesan cheese.

9. Pour the mixture into the skillet and scramble until set to your likeness, 2 minutes.

10. Between two chaffles, spoon half of the scrambled eggs and repeat with the second set of chaffles.

11. Serve afterward. Nutrition value per Servings:

Calories 387 Fat 22.52g Carbs 18g Protein 27.76g Sugar 2g

Peanut Butter Sandwich Chaffle

Servings: 1

Cooking Time: 15 Minutes

Ingredients:

For chaffle:

1 egg, lightly beaten

1/2 cup mozzarella cheese, shredded 1/4 tsp espresso powder 1 tbsp unsweetened chocolate chips

1   tbsp Swerve

2   tbsp unsweetened cocoa powder

For filling:

1 tbsp butter, softened 2 tbsp Swerve

3 tbsp creamy peanut butter

Directions:

1.   Preheat your waffle maker.

2.   In a bowl, whisk together egg, espresso powder, chocolate chips, Swerve, and cocoa powder.

3. Add mozzarella cheese and stir well.

4. Spray waffle maker with cooking spray.

5. Pour 1/2 of the batter in the hot waffle maker and cook for 3-4 minutes or until golden brown. Repeat with the remaining batter.

6. For filling: In a small bowl, stir together butter, Swerve, and peanut butter until smooth.

7. Once chaffles is cool, then spread filling mixture between two chaffle and place in the fridge for 10 minutes.

8. Cut chaffle sandwich in half and serve. Nutrition value:

Calories 70 Fat 16.1 g Carbohydrates 9.6 g Sugar 1.1 g Protein 8.2 g

Easter Morning Simple Chaffles

Servings:2

Cooking Time:5minutes

Ingredients:

1/2 cup egg whites

1 cup mozzarella cheese, melted

Directions:

1.   Switch on your square waffle maker. Spray with non-stick spray.

2.   Beat egg whites with beater, until fluffy and white.

3.   Add cheese and mix well.

4.   Pour batter in a waffle maker.

5.   Close the maker and cook for about 3 minutes.

6.   Repeat with the remaining batter.

7.   Remove chaffles from the maker.

8.   Serve hot and enjoy! Nutrition value per Servings:

Calories: 145 Fat: 9.4g Carbohydrates: 1g Sugar: 0.2g Protein: 14.3g

Apple Cinnamon Chaffles

Servings: 3

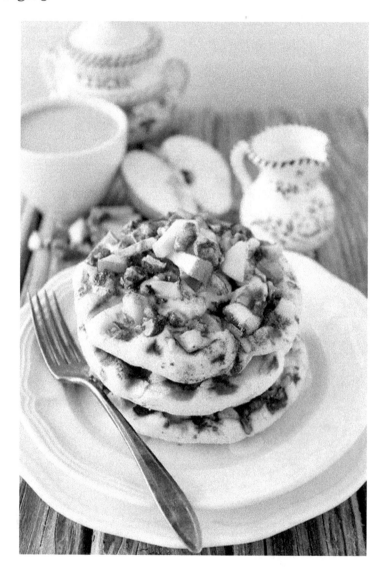

Cooking Time: 20 Minutes

Ingredients:

3 eggs, lightly beaten

1 cup mozzarella cheese, shredded ¼ cup apple, chopped

½ tsp monk fruit sweetener 1 ½ tsp cinnamon

¼ tsp baking powder, gluten-free 2 tbsp coconut flour

Directions:

1.   Preheat your waffle maker.

2.   Add remaining ingredients and stir until well combined.

3.   Spray waffle maker with cooking spray.

4.   Pour 1/3 of batter in the hot waffle maker and cook for minutes or until golden brown. Repeat with the remaining batter.

5.   Serve and enjoy. Nutrition value:

Calories 142 Fat 7.4 g Carbohydrates 9.7 g Sugar 3 g Protein 9.g

Churro Chaffle

Servings: 2

Cooking Time: 8 Minutes

Ingredients:

1   egg

½ cup mozzarella cheese, shredded ½ teaspoon cinnamon 2 tablespoons sweetener

Directions:

1.   Turn on your waffle iron.

2.   Beat the egg in a bowl.

3.   Stir in the cheese.

4.   Pour half of the mixture into the waffle maker.

5.   Cover the waffle iron.

6.   Cook for 4 minutes.

7.   While waiting, mix the cinnamon and sweetener in a bowl.

8.   Open the device and soak the waffle in the cinnamon mixture.

9.   Repeat the steps with the remaining batter. Nutrition value:

Calories 98 Fat 6.9g Carbohydrate 5.8g Protein 9.6g Sugars 0.4g

Super Easy Chocolate Chaffles

Servings: 2

Cooking Time:5 minutes

Ingredients:

1/4 cup unsweetened chocolate chips 1 egg

2   tbsps. almond flour

1/2 cup mozzarella cheese 1 tbsp. Greek yogurts

1/2 tsp. baking powder 1 tsp. stevia Directions:

1.   Switch on your square chaffle maker.

2.   Spray the waffle maker with cooking spray.

3.   Mix all recipe ingredients in a mixing bowl.

4.   Spoon batter in a greased waffle maker and make two chaffles.

5.   Once chaffles are cooked, remove from the maker.

6.   Serve with coconut cream, shredded chocolate, and nuts on top.

7.   Enjoy!

Nutrition value per Servings:

Calories: 145 Fat: 9.4g Carbohydrates: 1g Sugar: 0.2g Protein: 14.3g

Mini Keto Pizza

Servings: 2

Cooking Time: 15 Minutes

Ingredients:

1   egg

½ cup mozzarella cheese, shredded ¼ teaspoon basil

¼ teaspoon garlic powder 1 tablespoon almond flour

½ teaspoon baking powder

2   tablespoons reduced-carb pasta sauce 2 tablespoons mozzarella cheese Directions:

1.   Preheat your waffle maker.

2.   In a bowl, beat the egg.

3.   Stir in the ½ cup mozzarella cheese, basil, garlic powder, almond flour and baking powder.

4.   Add half of the mixture to your waffle maker.

5.   Cook for 4 minutes.

6.   Transfer to a baking sheet.

7.   Cook the second mini pizza.

8.   While both pizzas are on the baking sheet, spread the pasta sauce on top.

9.   Sprinkle the cheese on top.

10.   Bake in the oven until the cheese has melted. Nutrition value:

Calories 195 Fat 14 g Carbohydrate 4 g Protein 13 g Sugars 1 g

Keto Chaffle With Almond Flour

Servings: 2

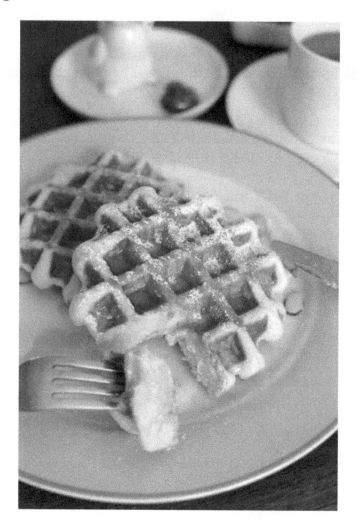

Cooking Time: 8 Minutes

Ingredients:

1 egg, beaten

½ cup cheddar cheese, shredded 1 tablespoon almond flour

Directions:

1.   Turn on your waffle maker.

2.   Mix all the ingredients in a bowl.

3.   Pour half of the batter into the waffle maker.

4.   Close the device and cook for minutes.

5.   Remove from the waffle maker.

6.   Let sit for 2 to 3 minutes.

7.   Repeat the steps with the remaining batter. Nutrition value:

Calories 145 Fat 11 g Carbohydrate 1 g Protein 10 g Total Sugars 1 g

Chaffles With Caramelized Apples And Yogurt

Servings: 2

Cooking Time: 10 Minutes

Ingredients:

1 tablespoon unsalted butter

1 tablespoon golden brown sugar

1   Granny Smith apple, cored and thinly sliced 1 pinch salt

2   whole-grain frozen waffles, toasted

1/2 cup mozzarella cheese, shredded

1/4 cup Yoplait® Original French Vanilla yogurt

Directions:

Melt the butter in a large skillet over medium-high heat until starting to

brown. Add mozzarella cheese and stir well.

Add the sugar, apple slices, salt, and cook, stirring frequently, until apples are softened and tender, about 6 to 9 minutes.

Put one warm waffle each on a plate, top each with yogurt and apples. Serve warm.

Nutrition value:

Calories: 240 Fat: 10.4 g Carbohydrate: 33.8 g Protein: 4.7 g

Keto Chaffle With Ice-Cream

Servings: 2

Cooking Time: 5 Minutes

Ingredients:

1 egg

1/2 cup cheddar cheese, shredded 1 tbsp. almond flour

½ tsp. baking powder. FOR SERVING

1/2 cup heavy cream

1   tbsp. keto chocolate chips. 2 oz. raspberries

2   oz. blueberries

Directions:

1.   Preheat your minutesi waffle maker according to the manufacturer's Directions.

2.   Mix chaffle ingredients in a small bowl and make minutesi chaffles.

3.   For an ice-cream ball, mix cream and chocolate chips in a bowl and pour

this mixture in 2 silicone molds.

4.   Freeze the ice-cream balls in a freezer for about 2-hours.

5.   For serving, set ice-cream ball on chaffle.

6.   Top with berries and enjoy! Nutrition value per Servings:

Calories: 145 Fat: 9.4g Carbohydrates: 1g Sugar: 0.2g Protein:
14.3g

Chaffle Tortilla

Servings: 2

Cooking Time: 8 Minutes

Ingredients:

1 egg

½ cup cheddar cheese, shredded 1 teaspoon baking powder

4 tablespoons almond flour

¼ teaspoon garlic powder

1 tablespoon almond milk Homemade salsa Sour cream

Jalapeno pepper, chopped

Directions:

1.   Preheat your waffle maker.

2.   Beat the egg in a bowl.

3.   Stir in the cheese, baking powder, flour, garlic powder and almond milk.

4.   Pour half of the batter into the waffle maker.

5.   Cover and cook for 4 minutes.

6. Open and transfer to a plate. Let cool for 2 minutes.

7. Do the same for the remaining batter.

8. Top the waffle with salsa, sour cream and jalapeno pepper.

9. Roll the waffle. Nutrition value:

Calories 225 Fat 17.6g Carbohydrate 6g Protein 11.3g Sugars 1.9g

Chicken Quesadilla Chaffle

Servings: 2

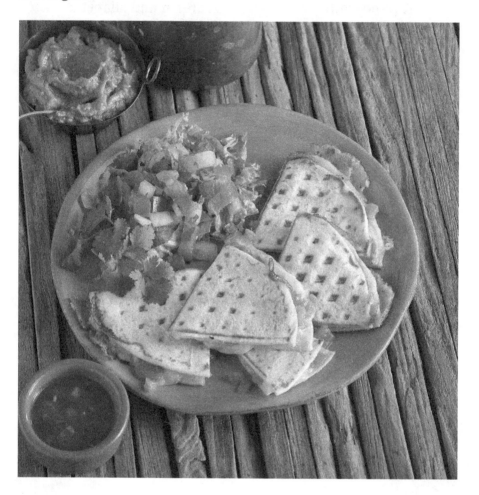

Cooking Time: 14 Minutes

Ingredients:

1 egg, beaten

¼ tsp taco seasoning

1/3 cup finely grated cheddar cheese 1/3 cup cooked chopped chicken Directions:

1.   Preheat the waffle iron.

2.   In a medium bowl, mix the eggs, taco seasoning, and cheddar cheese. Add the chicken and combine well.

3.   Open the iron, lightly grease with cooking spray and pour in half of the mixture.

4.   Close the iron and cook until brown and crispy, 7 minutes.

5.   Remove the chaffle onto a plate and set aside.

6.   Make another chaffle using the remaining mixture.

7.   Serve afterward. Nutrition value per Servings:

Calories 314 Fat 20.64g Carbs 5.71g Protein 16.74g

Chocolate Chip Chaffle

Servings: 2

Cooking Time: 8 Minutes

Ingredients:

1 egg

½ teaspoon coconut flour

¼ teaspoon baking powder 1 teaspoon sweetener

1 tablespoon heavy whipping cream 1 tablespoon chocolate chips
Directions:

1.   Preheat your waffle maker.

2.   Beat the egg in a bowl.

3.   Stir in the flour, baking powder, sweetener and cream.

4.   Pour half of the mixture into the waffle maker.

5.   Sprinkle the chocolate chips on top and close.

6.   Cook for 4 minutes.

7.   Remove the chaffle and put on a plate.

8.   Do the same procedure with the remaining batter.

Nutrition value:

Calories 146 Fat 10 g Carbohydrate 5 g Protein 6 g Sugars 1 g

Cheese Garlic Chaffle

Servings: 2

Cooking Time: 8 Minutes

Ingredients:

Chaffle 1 egg

1 teaspoon cream cheese

½ cup mozzarella cheese, shredded ½ teaspoon garlic powder 1 teaspoon Italian seasoning

Topping

1   tablespoon butter

½ teaspoon garlic powder

½ teaspoon Italian seasoning

2   tablespoon mozzarella cheese, shredded

Directions:

1.   Plug in your waffle maker to preheat.

2.   Preheat your oven to 350 degrees F.

3.   In a bowl, combine all the chaffle ingredients.

4. Cook in the waffle maker for minutes per chaffle.

5. Transfer to a baking pan.

6. Spread butter on top of each chaffle.

7. Sprinkle garlic powder and Italian seasoning on top.

8. Top with mozzarella cheese.

9. Bake until the cheese has melted. Nutrition value:

Calories141 Fat 13 g Carbohydrate 2.6g

Lemon And Vanilla Chaffle

Servings:4

Cooking Time:7-9 Minutes

Ingredients:

Batter 4 eggs

4 ounces ricotta cheese

2 teaspoons vanilla extract

2 tablespoons fresh lemon juice Zest of ½ lemon 6 tablespoons stevia

5 tablespoons coconut flour

½ teaspoon baking powder Other

2 tablespoons butter to brush the waffle maker

Directions:

1.   Preheat the waffle maker.

2.   Add the eggs and ricotta cheese to a bowl and stir with a wire whisk until just combined.

3.   Add the vanilla extract, lemon juice, lemon zest, and stevia and mix until combined.

4.   Stir in the coconut flour and baking powder until combined.

5.   Brush the heated waffle maker with butter and add a few tablespoons of the batter.

6.   Close the lid and cook for about 7-8 minutes depending on your waffle maker.

7.   Serve and enjoy. Nutrition value per Servings:

Calories 200, fat 13.4 g, carbs 9 g, sugar 0.9 g, Protein 10.2 g

Christmas Smoothie With Chaffles

Servings: 2

Cooking Time: 10 Minutes

Ingredients:

1   cupcoconutmilk

2   tbsps. almonds chopped ¼ cup cherries 1 pinch sea salt

1/4 cup ice cubes FOR TOPPING:

2 oz. keto chocolate chips 2 oz. cherries

2 minutesi chaffles

2 scoop heavy cream, frozen

Directions:

1.   Add almond milk, almonds, cherries, salt and ice in a blender, blend for 2 minutes until smooth and fluffy.

2.   Pour the smoothie into glasses.

3.   Top with one scoop heavy cream, chocolate chips, cherries and chaffle in each glass.

4.   Serve and enjoy! Nutrition value per Servings:

Calories: 145 Fat: 9.4g Carbohydrates: 1g Sugar: 0.2g Protein: 14.3g

Raspberry And Chocolate Chaffle

Servings:4

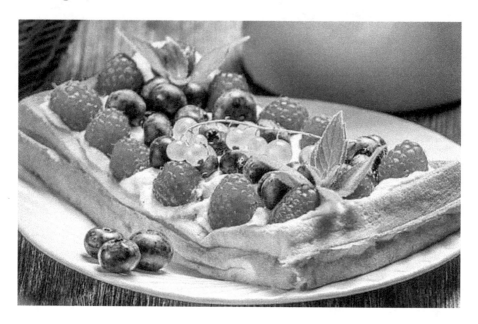

Cooking Time:7-9 Minutes

Ingredients:

Batter

4 eggs

2 ounces cream cheese, softened

2 ounces sour cream

1 teaspoon vanilla extract

5 tablespoons almond flour ¼ cup cocoa powder 1½ teaspoons baking powder

2 ounces fresh or frozen raspberries

2 tablespoons butter to brush the waffle maker Fresh sprigs of mint to garnish

Directions:

1.   Preheat the waffle maker.

2.   Add the eggs, cream cheese and sour cream to a bowl and stir with a wire whisk until combined.

3.   Add the vanilla extract and mix until combined.

4.   Stir in the almond flour, cocoa powder, and baking powder and mix until combined.

5.   Add the raspberries and stir until combined.

6.   Brush the heated waffle maker with butter and add a few tablespoons of the batter.

7.   Close the lid and cook for about 8 minutes depending on your waffle maker.

8.   Serve with fresh sprigs of mint. Nutrition value per Servings:

Calories 270, fat 23 g, carbs 8.g, sugar 1.3 g, Protein 10.2 g

Pumkpin Chaffle With Maple Syrup

Servings: 2

Cooking Time: 16 Minutes

Ingredients:

2 eggs, beaten

½ cup mozzarella cheese, shredded 1 teaspoon coconut flour

¾ teaspoon baking powder

¾ teaspoon pumpkin pie spice 2 teaspoons pureed pumpkin

4 teaspoons heavy whipping cream ½ teaspoon vanilla Pinch salt

2 teaspoons maple syrup (sugar-free)

Directions:

1.   Turn your waffle maker on.

2.   Mix all the ingredients except maple syrup in a large bowl.

3.   Pour half of the batter into the waffle maker.

4.   Close and cook for minutes.

5. Transfer to a plate to cool for 2 minutes.

6. Repeat the steps with the remaining mixture.

7. Drizzle the maple syrup on top of the chaffles before serving. Nutrition value:

Calories 201 Fat 15 g Carbohydrate 4 g Protein 12 g Sugars 1 g

Turkey Bbq Sauce Chaffle

Servings:4

Cooking Time:8-10 Minutes

Ingredients:

Batter

½ pound ground turkey meat 3 eggs

1 cup grated Swiss cheese

¼ cup cream cheese

¼ cup BBQ sauce

1   teaspoon dried oregano Salt and pepper to taste

2   cloves garlic, minced

2 tablespoons butter to brush the waffle maker ¼ cup BBQ sauce for serving 2 tablespoons freshly chopped parsley for garnish

Directions:

1.   Preheat the waffle maker.

2. Add the ground turkey, eggs, grated Swiss cheese, cream cheese, BBQ sauce, dried oregano, salt and pepper, and minced garlic to a bowl.

3. Mix everything until combined and batter forms.

4. Brush the heated waffle maker with butter and add a few tablespoons of

the batter.

5. Close the lid and cook for about 8-10 minutes depending on your waffle maker.

6. Serve each chaffle with a tablespoon of BBQ sauce and a sprinkle of freshly chopped parsley.

Nutrition value per Servings:

Calories 365, fat 23.g, carbs 13.7 g, sugar 8.8 g, Protein 23.5 g

Strawberry Cream Sandwich Chaffles

Servings: 2

Cooking Time: 6 Minutes

Ingredients:

Chaffles

1 large organic egg, beaten

½ cup mozzarella cheese, shredded finely Filling

4 teaspoons heavy cream

2 tablespoons powdered erythritol 1 teaspoon fresh lemon juice
Pinch of fresh lemon zest, grated

2 fresh strawberries, hulled and sliced

Directions:

1.   Preheat a mini waffle iron and then grease it.

2.   For chaffles: in a small bowl, add the egg and mozzarella
cheese and stir to combine.

3.   Place half of the mixture into preheated waffle iron and
cook for about 2- minutes.

4.   Repeat with the remaining mixture.

5.   Meanwhile, for filling: in a bowl, Place all the ingredients except the strawberry slices and with a hand mixer, beat until well combined.

6.   Serve each chaffle with cream mixture and strawberry slices. Nutrition value:

Calories 95 Fat 5 g Carbs 1.7 g Fiber 0.3 g Sugar 0.9 g Protein 5.5 g

Ham Sandwich Chaffles

Servings: 2

Cooking Time: 8 Minutes

Ingredients:

1   organic egg, beaten

½ cup Monterrey Jack cheese, shredded 1 teaspoon coconut flour

Pinch of garlic powder Filling

2   sugar-free ham slices 1 small tomato, sliced 2 lettuce leaves Directions:

1.   Preheat a mini waffle iron and then grease it.

2.   For chaffles: In a medium bowl, put all ingredients and with a fork, mix until well combined. Place

half of the mixture into preheated waffle iron and cook for about 3-4 minutes.

3.   Repeat with the remaining mixture.

4.   Serve each chaffle with filling ingredients. Nutrition value:

Calories 100 Fat 8.7 g Carbs 5.5 g Fiber 1.8 g Sugar 1.5 g Protein 13.9 g

Chicken Sandwich Chaffles

Servings: 2

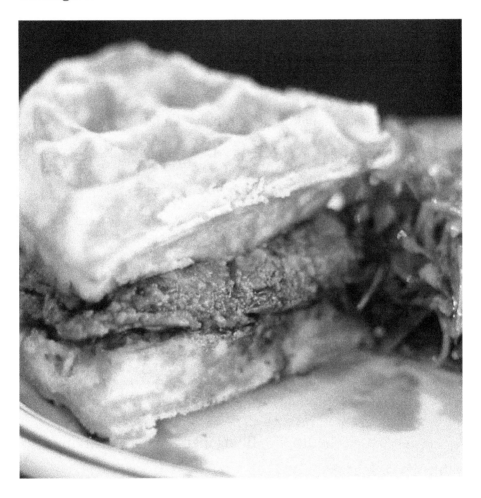

Cooking Time: 8 Minutes

Ingredients:

Chaffles

1 large organic egg, beaten

½ cup cheddar cheese, shredded

Pinch of salt and ground black pepper

Filling

1 (6-ounce) cooked chicken breast, halved 2 lettuce leaves

¼ of small onion, sliced

1   small tomato, sliced

Directions:

1.   Preheat a mini waffle iron and then grease it.

2.   For chaffles: In a medium bowl, put all ingredients and with a fork, mix until well combined.Place half of the mixture into preheated waffle iron and cook for about 3-4 minutes.

3.   Repeat with the remaining mixture.

4.   Serve each chaffle with filling ingredients. Nutrition value:

Calories 159 Fat 14.1 g Carbs 3.3 g Sugar 2 g Protein 28.7 g

Pork Chaffles On Pan

Servings:4

Cooking Time:5minutes

Ingredients:

1 cup pork, minutesced

1 egg

½ cup chopped parsley 1 cup cheddar cheese pinch of salt

1 tbsp. avocado oil

Directions:

1. Heat your nonstick pan over medium heat.

2. In a small bowl, mix pork, parsley, egg, and cheese

3. Grease pan with avocado oil.

4. Once the pan is hot, pour 2 tbsps. pork batter and cook for about 1-2 minutes.

5. Flip and cook for another 1-2 minutes.

6. Once chaffle is brown, remove from pan.

7. Serve BBQ sauce on top and enjoy! Nutrition value per Servings:

Calories 178 Fat 15.5g Carbohydrate 1.9g Protein 5.4g Sugars 0.6g

Oven-Baked Chaffles

Servings:10

Cooking Time:5 Minutes

Ingredients:

3 eggs

2 cups mozzarella cheese

¼ cup coconut flour 1 tsp. baking powder 1 tbsp. coconut oil

1 tsp stevia

1 tbsp. coconut cream

Directions:

1. Preheat oven on 4000 F.

2. Mix all ingredients in a bowl.

3. Pour batter in silicon waffle mold and set it on a baking tray.

4. Bake chaffles in an oven for about 10-15 minutes.

5. Once cooked, remove from oven

6. Serve hot with coffee and enjoy! Nutrition value per Servings:

Calories 188 Fat 17.5g Carbohydrate 2.6g Protein 8.4g Sugars 0.6g

Pumpkin Pecan Chaffle

Servings: 2

Cooking Time: 10 Minutes

Ingredients:

2 tbsp toasted pecans (chopped) 2 tbsp almond flour

1 tbsp pumpkin puree

½ tsp pumpkin spice

½ cup grated mozzarella cheese

1 tsp granulated swerve sweetener 1 egg

½ tsp nutmeg

½ tsp vanilla extract

½ tsp baking powder

Directions:

1. Plug the waffle maker to preheat it and spray it with a non-stick spray.

2. In a mixing bowl, combine the almond flour, baking powder, pumpkin spice, swerve, cheese and nutmeg.

3. In another mixing bowl, whisk together the pumpkin puree egg and vanilla extract.

4. Pour the egg mixture into the flour mixture and mix until the ingredients are well combined.

5. Pour an appropriate amount of the batter into the waffle maker and spread out the batter to the edges to cover all the holes on the waffle maker.

6. Close the waffle maker and cook for about 5 minutes or according to your waffle maker's settings.

7. After the cooking cycle, use a silicone or plastic utensil to remove the chaffle from the waffle maker.

8. Repeat step 5 to 7 until you have cooked all the batter into chaffles.

9. Serve warm and top with whipped cream. Enjoy!!! Nutrition value per Servings:

Calories 178 Fat 5.5g Carbohydrate 0.6g Protein 6.4g Sugars 0.6g

French Toast Chaffle Sticks

Servings: 8

Cooking Time: 40 Minutes

Ingredients:

6 organic eggs

2 cups mozzarella cheese, shredded ¼ cup coconut flour 2 tablespoons powdered erythritol

1 teaspoon ground cinnamon 1 tablespoon butter, melted

Directions:

1.   Preheat your oven to 350°F and line a large baking sheet with a greased piece of foil.

2.   Preheat a waffle iron and then grease it.

3.   In a bowl, add 4 eggs and beat well.

4.   Add the cheese, coconut flour, erythritol and ½ teaspoon of cinnamon and mix until well combined.

5.   Place ¼ of the mixture into preheated waffle iron and cook for about 6-8 minutes.

6.   Repeat with the remaining mixture.

7.   Set the chaffles aside to cool.

8.   Cut each chaffle into 4 strips.

9.   In a large bowl, add the remaining eggs and cinnamon and beat until well combined.

10.   Dip the chaffle sticks in the egg mixture evenly.

11.   Arrange the chaffle sticks onto the prepared baking sheet in a single layer.

12.   Bake for about 10 minutes.

13.   Remove the baking sheet from oven and brush the top of each stick with the melted butter.

14.   Flip the stick and bake for about 6-8 minutes.

15.   Serve immediately.

Nutrition value:

Calories 96 Fat 6.3 g Carbs 3.2 g Fiber 1.7 g Sugar 0.3 g Protein 6.7 g

Fruity Vegan Chaffles

Servings Provided: 2

Nutritional Facts - Per Serving:

- Net Carbohydrates: 1.6 grams

- Calories: 130

- Protein: 10.1 grams

- Fats: 42.3 grams

Ingredients Needed:

- Chia seeds (1 tbsp.)

- Warm water (2 tbsp.)

- Low-carb vegan cheese (.25 cup)

- Greek yogurt (2 tbsp.)

- Strawberry puree (2 tbsp.)

- Salt (a pinch)

Preparation Directions:

1. Warm the mini waffle maker using the med–high temperature setting. Lightly grease the grids.

2. Combine the water and chia seeds to soak 3-4 minutes to thicken.

3. When it's ready, stir in the rest of the fixings.

4. Pour the batter into the waffle maker's center and cook each batch for three to five minutes.

5. Serve with the berries on top.

Servings:

Calories 208 Fat 13.5g Carbohydrate 0.7g Protein 8.2g Sugars 0.6g

Bacon Jalapeno Popper Chaffle

Servings: 3

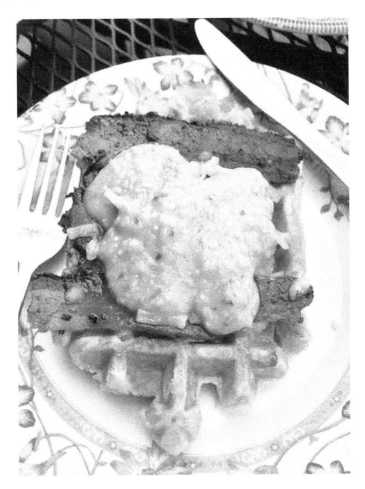

Cooking Time: 10 Minutes

Ingredients:

4 slices bacon (diced) 3 eggs

3 tbsp coconut flour 1 tsp baking powder

¼ tsp salt

½ tsp oregano

A pinch of onion powder A pinch of garlic powder

½ cup cream cheese

1   cup shredded cheddar cheese

2   jalapeno pepper (deseeded and chopped) ½ cup sour cream

Directions:

1.   Plug the waffle maker to preheat it and spray it with a non-stick cooking spray.

2.   Heat a frying pan over medium to high heat. Add the bacon and saute until the bacon is brown and crispy.

3.   Use a slotted spoon to transfer the bacon to a paper towel lined plate to drain.

4.   In a mixing bowl, combine the coconut flour, baking powder, salt, oregano, onion and garlic.

5.   In another mixing bowl, whisk together the egg and cream cheese until well combined.

6.   Add the cheddar cheese and mix. Pour in the flour mixture and mix until you form a smooth batter.

7.   Pour an appropriate amount of the batter into the waffle maker and spread it to the edges to cover all the holes on the waffle maker.

8.   Close the waffle maker and cook for about 5 minutes or according to waffle maker's settings.

9.   After the cooking cycle, use a plastic or silicone utensil to remove the chaffle from the waffle maker.

10.   Repeat step 7 to 9 until you have cooked all the batter into chaffles.

11.   Serve warm and top with sour cream, crispy bacon and jalapeno slices. Nutrition value per Servings:

Calories 208 Fat 13.5g Carbohydrate 0.7g Protein 8.2g Sugars 0.6g

Apple Pie Chaffle

Servings: 2

Cooking Time: 6 Minutes

Ingredients:

1 egg (beaten)

1 tbsp almond flour

1 big apple (finely chopped) 1 tbsp heavy whipping cream 1 tsp cinnamon

1 tbsp granulated swerve

½ tsp vanilla extract

1/3 cup mozzarella cheese Topping:

¼ tbsp sugar free maple syrup

Directions:

1.   Plug the waffle maker and preheat it. Spray it with non-stick spray.

2.   In a large mixing bowl, combine the swerve, almond flour, mozzarella, cinnamon and chopped apple.

3.   Add the eggs, vanilla extract and heavy whipping cream. Mix until all the ingredients are well combined.

4.   Fill the waffle maker with the batter and spread out the batter to the waffle maker's edges to all the holes on it.

5.   Close the waffle maker's lid and cook for about 4 minutes or according to waffle maker's settings.

6.   After the cooking cycle, remove the chaffle from the waffle maker with a plastic or silicone utensil.

7.   Repeat step 4 to 6 until you have cooked all the batter into chaffles.

8.   Serve and top with maple syrup. Nutrition value per Servings:

Calories 228 Fat 17.5g Carbohydrate 2.7g Protein 5.2g Sugars 2g

CPSIA information can be obtained
at www.ICGtesting.com
Printed in the USA
BVHW061032220321
603178BV00004B/352